Diabetes-free Pregnancy: Nourish, Energise, Thrive.

Diabetes-free Pregnancy: Nourish, Energise and Thrive

Ruby Gumbi-Edwards

Published by Ruby G Edwards, 2023.

While every precaution has been taken in the preparation of this book, the publisher assumes no responsibility for errors or omissions, or for damages resulting from the use of the information contained herein.

DIABETES-FREE PREGNANCY: NOURISH, ENERGISE AND THRIVE

First edition. July 26, 2023.

Copyright © 2023 Ruby Gumbi-Edwards.

ISBN: 979-8223593232

Written by Ruby Gumbi-Edwards.

Table of Contents

Dedication

My father, a gymnast and Marshal Arts Coach, taught me nutrition and anatomy when I was three.

He taught me to work hard as a gymnast...He taught me to only eat natural foods. My home was candy-free. For sweet cravings, we only ate fresh fruit, unsulphured dried fruit, and home-made chocolate with cocoa.

In every gymnastics class, my father said, "Never forget...you are what you eat!" - I learned this. It became my life code.

In a sugar-filled fast food world, more than ever. Sugar kills. It's everywhere, including kids' food.

I dedicate this book to my father, who inspired my healthy lifestyle. Second, to my late mother who made the healthiest and tastiest meals. Finally, I dedicate this book to all women, wishing them a diabetes-free life full of health and happiness. My father, a gymnast and Marshal Arts Coach, taught me gymnastics from age three.

He taught me to work hard as a gymnast...He taught me to only eat natural foods. My home was candy-free. For sweet cravings, we only ate fresh fruit, unsulphured dried fruit, and homemade chocolate with cacao.

In every gymnastics class, my father said, "Never forget...you are what you eat!" - I learned this. It became my life code.

In a sugar-filled fast food world, more than ever. Sugar kills. It's everywhere, including in children's food.

I dedicate this book to my father, who inspired my healthy lifestyle. Second, my late mother, who cooked the healthiest and tastiest meals. Finally, I dedicate this book to all women, globally, wishing you all a diabetes-free life full of health, happiness and prosperity.

Contents

Foreword

Disclaimer: I am not a doctor. Reading this book should encourage you to take good care of yourself and part of doing that is to ensure you have a good doctor, who you like and can rely upon. So consult with your doctor for any clinical diagnoses.

I became a gymnast almost as soon as I could walk, as my father was a Physical Educationist specialising in coaching gymnastics. He was also a Personal Trainer and school Physical Training Instructor. So I grew up as a horse rider, ballet, and contemporary dancer, and as a gymnast. My father was the Founder of the Soweto Gymnastics Association. A member of The South African Gymnastics Association... and my very own personal gymnastics coach, personal trainer, and nutritionist. The gymnasium became my second home. From Monday to Friday, I spent most of my out-of-school hours in the gym, practicing and sometimes assisting my father in training junior gymnasts. I also performed at schools... before and after the motivational speaking sessions my Father gave to governing school bodies, teachers, and pupils. He always stressed the importance of a natural diet and the nutritional necessity to develop a healthy body and mind.

Teaching how nutrition was The Creator's design, tried and tested mechanism from mother nature, that helps prevent and even cure disease. Early on, exercise became the cornerstone of my lifestyle.

And in our family, we only ate and drank natural foods and beverages, and took organic supplements, which became a code I lived by. As my father encouraged me to read and learn from world-renowned health professionals, which became one of my great commitments.

Following nature's code of conduct has kept me away from needing traditional clinical treatment to date... and so I hope this book will help you to do the same.

One final thought...Go swimming!!!

The baby grows comfortably in the water of the mother's womb. So a baby who starts swimming at 6 months can become a great swimmer by about 18 months. Or even earlier. Being a swimmer is a life-changing experience. You just need water to access a world of fabulous physical exercise that is also a wonderful meditation. So give your baby a brilliant life skill that will help your child be fit and strong. Calm, confident, and happy... for the rest of their life! Swimming, especially at sea, is like being in your mother's womb again, feeling safe. It will change your life!

Much Love, Ruby.

Introduction:

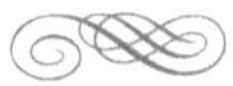

Your body is your number one nutritionist. Nature and food are your number one medicine. Exercise is your muscles and body toner. Prayer nourishes your soul and meditation calms the state of being.

Listen to your body because, through it, you will always know how well or unwell you feel. Because the body is the antenna with all the senses; sight, hearing, smell, taste, and touch which function in conjunction with the subconscious mind.

"When your health is absent wisdom cannot reveal itself. Art cannot manifest. Strength cannot fight. Wealth becomes useless and intelligence cannot be applied. Invest in your health today!"

~ Herophilus.

Chapter 1: Pregnancy

The butterfly metamorphosis connection to pregnancy

The butterfly metamorphosis entails distinct stages of; egg, caterpillar, chrysalis, and butterfly, which can serve as an analogy to the process of a woman wishing to have a baby in terms of personal growth and transformation.

Pregnancy and metamorphosis manifestation connection:

A woman's desire for a baby is similar to the butterfly's life cycle starting with an egg of a butterfly. A woman's journey toward motherhood often begins in her imagination with the dream to have a baby. This stage represents the initial longing and the potential for new life.

A woman preparing for pregnancy may focus on her health, lifestyle choices, and seeking medical advice to optimise her chances of conceiving and creating an ideal environment for the baby's development. Quite similar to preconception and preparation in the caterpillar stage.

The butterfly larva grows and develops, consuming resources to fuel its transformation. The nurturing stage, a pregnant woman provides a safe and nourishing environment for her growing foetus. During this stage, the woman's body goes through several changes to support the baby's growth. Likewise, just as the chrysalis protects and nurtures the developing butterfly.

The chrysalis stage symbolises the period of pregnancy.

The birth of new life. Finally, the butterfly emerges from the chrysalis, representing the birth of a baby. This stage symbolises the joy and fulfillment of the woman's journey to motherhood, as a new life is welcomed into the world.

The butterfly transformation can be seen as a metaphor for human pregnancy in several ways:

- **Transformation:** Pregnancy is a transformational journey for a woman, similar to the miraculous metamorphosis of a butterfly from an egg to a caterpillar, then a chrysalis, and finally emerging as a magnificent butterfly. As she prepares to give birth, she undergoes significant physical, emotional, and psychological changes.

- **Growth and Development:** Just as a caterpillar grows and changes inside its chrysalis, a baby develops and grows inside the womb throughout pregnancy. Both processes include a remarkable evolution of growth, organ development, and the establishment of distinguishing characteristics.

- **Time and Patience:** The butterfly metamorphosis process takes time and requires patience. Similarly, pregnancy is a journey that lasts several months, during which the unborn child steadily matures and prepares for life outside the womb. It teaches us about perseverance and embracing life's natural course.

- **Beauty and Wonder:** The emergence of a butterfly from its chrysalis is a breathtaking sight. Similarly, a baby's birth is a joyful and beautiful miracle. Both signify new beginnings, the start of a new life, and an appreciation of the spectacular beauty that exists on our planet.

• **Symbol of Transformation and Renewal:** Butterflies are often seen as symbols of renewal and transformation. They represent the idea of growth and the emergence of something beautiful. In the same way, pregnancy represents a woman's transformative journey, which culminates in the birth of a child and the beginning of a new chapter.

Women's wish, dream, and desire to have a baby

This sensation indicates her mental preparation to become a mother. It is infinite intelligence, the Creative Spirit manifesting its power through you.

Becoming a mother expresses one of the primary rules that govern our lives. Along with the Law of Attraction, the Law of Gestation is one of the most important natural laws that humans try to understand.

When a single woman is desperately trying to conceive, a man appears out of nowhere, she falls deeply in love, and she conceives. Because The Law of Attraction has the power to bring our deepest hopes and wishes to fruition when we make a faithful vow to the universe. Bringing the things we need into our life at the exact moment we need them.

Every day of my life I use the power of this phenomenon to remind myself of the profound mystery and power of life. Especially when, despite its seeming simplicity, life is frequently complex.

So I hope that this book will assist you in learning more by simplifying various facts and ideas. Helping to broaden your mind in the nicest possible way. And I thank you for allowing me to share my experiences, thoughts, and viewpoints on the wonders of life... Enjoy!

What is Pregnancy?

Pregnancy lasts around 40 weeks, divided into three trimesters;

Pregnancy is the condition of bearing an embryo or foetus inside the female reproductive system. It occurs when a sperm fertilises an egg through sexual intercourse or through assisted reproductive methods, such as in vitro fertilisation (IVF).

The first trimester is distinguished by the foetus' early formation and development, whilst the second and third trimesters are distinguished by the foetus' continued growth and maturation. During pregnancy, a woman's body undergoes hormonal and physiological changes in order to encourage the development of the baby and prepare for childbirth.

Although pregnancy symptoms and signs vary, common early warning indicators include missed periods, sensitive breasts, tiredness, nausea, and excessive urination. Other pregnancy symptoms, including as weight gain, an enlarging belly, stretch marks, and changes in the woman's body structure, may appear as the pregnancy progresses.

Regular prenatal care is vital for tracking your own health and the growth of the baby, as well as your own during pregnancy. Regular check-ups, medical exams, and meetings with medical specialists are all part of ensuring a safe pregnancy and dealing with any potential challenges or concerns.

Childbirth is the most advanced stage of pregnancy, in which the baby is born either through a vaginal birth or cesarean section based on a variety of factors such as the mother's health, the baby's position, and any potential complexities.

After childbirth, the postpartum period begins, during which the mother's body continues to change and adapt while she cares for her newborn.

Consult with a healthcare professional for personal tailored guidance and support during your pregnancy.

Pregnancy is a complex and unique experience for each woman, bringing both joy and trials. The mother's body undergoes additional changes and modifications during the postpartum while caring for her newborn.

It's important to note that pregnancy is a complex, challenging, and a unique experience for each woman, it can bring both joy and challenges. It is advisable to consult with healthcare professionals for personalised guidance and assistance throughout your pregnancy journey.

Tips to cope with the body change during pregnancy

Dealing with the physical changes during pregnancy can vary for each woman, as everyone's experience and comfort levels differ. However, here are some general tips to help women cope with the changes in their physique during pregnancy:

- **Embrace the changes:** Pregnancy is a beautiful and life-changing experience. It's critical to embrace and appreciate the changes happening to your body as it nurtures and grows another life. Remind yourself that these changes are temporary and a natural part of the process.

If you're struggling with body image or finding it challenging to cope with the changes, consider speaking to an elder, or a close friend who comes out of pregnancy in a good way, overall. Or speak to a healthcare professional or counselor you trust to give you good advice and provide additional guidance and support.

• Symbol of Transformation and Renewal: Butterflies are often seen as symbols of renewal and transformation. They represent the idea of growth and the emergence of something beautiful. In the same way, pregnancy represents a woman's transformative journey, which culminates in the birth of a child and the beginning of a new chapter.

Women's wish, dream, and desire to have a baby

This sensation indicates her mental preparation to become a mother. It is infinite intelligence, the Creative Spirit manifesting its power through you.

Becoming a mother expresses one of the primary rules that govern our lives. Along with the Law of Attraction, the Law of Gestation is one of the most important natural laws that humans try to understand.

When a single woman is desperately trying to conceive, a man appears out of nowhere, she falls deeply in love, and she conceives. Because The Law of Attraction has the power to bring our deepest hopes and wishes to fruition when we make a faithful vow to the universe. Bringing the things we need into our life at the exact moment we need them.

Every day of my life I use the power of this phenomenon to remind myself of the profound mystery and power of life. Especially when, despite its seeming simplicity, life is frequently complex.

So I hope that this book will assist you in learning more by simplifying various facts and ideas. Helping to broaden your mind in the nicest possible way. And I thank you for allowing me to share my experiences, thoughts, and viewpoints on the wonders of life... Enjoy!

What is Pregnancy?

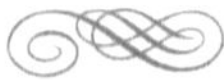

Pregnancy lasts around 40 weeks, divided into three trimesters;

Pregnancy is the condition of bearing an embryo or foetus inside the female reproductive system. It occurs when a sperm fertilises an egg through sexual intercourse or through assisted reproductive methods, such as in vitro fertilisation (IVF).

The first trimester is distinguished by the foetus' early formation and development, whilst the second and third trimesters are distinguished by the foetus' continued growth and maturation. During pregnancy, a woman's body undergoes hormonal and physiological changes in order to encourage the development of the baby and prepare for childbirth.

Although pregnancy symptoms and signs vary, common early warning indicators include missed periods, sensitive breasts, tiredness, nausea, and excessive urination. Other pregnancy symptoms, including as weight gain, an enlarging belly, stretch marks, and changes in the woman's body structure, may appear as the pregnancy progresses.

Regular prenatal care is vital for tracking your own health and the growth of the baby, as well as your own during pregnancy. Regular check-ups, medical exams, and meetings with medical specialists are all part of ensuring a safe pregnancy and dealing with any potential challenges or concerns.

Childbirth is the most advanced stage of pregnancy, in which the baby is born either through a vaginal birth or cesarean section based on a variety of factors such as the mother's health, the baby's position, and any potential complexities.

Consult with a healthcare professional for personalised and tailored guidance, and support during your pregnancy.

Pregnancy is a complex and unique experience for each woman, bringing both joy and trials. The mother's body undergoes additional changes and modifications during the postpartum while caring for her newborn.

It's important to note that pregnancy is a complex, challenging, and a unique experience for each woman, it can bring both joy and challenges. It is advisable to consult with healthcare professionals for personalised guidance and assistance throughout your pregnancy journey.

Tips to cope with the body change during pregnancy

Dealing with the physical changes during pregnancy can vary for each woman, as everyone's experience and comfort levels differ. However, here are some general tips to help women cope with the changes in their physique during pregnancy:

- **Embrace the changes:** Pregnancy is a beautiful and life-changing experience. It's critical to embrace and appreciate the changes happening to your body as it nurtures and grows another life. Remind yourself that these changes are temporary and a natural part of the process.

If you're struggling with body image or finding it challenging to cope with the changes, consider speaking to an elder, a close friend who comes out of pregnancy in a good way, overall. Or speak to a healthcare professional or counselor you trust to give you good advice and provide additional guidance and support.

After childbirth, the postpartum period begins, during which the mother's body continues to change and adapt while she cares for her newborn.

- **Wear comfortable clothing:** As your body stretches, it is critical to wear comfortable clothing that supports and accepts your developing tummy. Maternity apparel designed specifically for pregnant women can be advantageous in terms of comfort and growth.

- **Communicate with your partner:** Discuss your feelings and concerns with your partner, openly. They can offer understanding, support, and reassurance during this transformative time. Sharing your experiences and discussing any body image concerns can help foster a supportive environment.

Remember, every woman's pregnancy experience is unique, and it's essential to be kind to yourself and prioritise your physical and emotional well-being.

- **Stay active:** If your doctor agrees, you should continue to engage in regular physical activity during your pregnancy to promote both your physical and mental well-being. Good low-impact exercises include; walking, swimming, prenatal yoga, and aerobics. These exercises can help tone your muscles, promote circulation, relieve discomfort, and improve your overall health.

- **Take care of your posture:** It's common to notice changes in your posture as your belly expands, which can cause backaches and discomfort.

Maintain good posture by sitting and standing upright, sleeping on supportive pillows, and wearing supportive shoes. Prenatal exercises that target core and back muscles can also be beneficial.

- **Prioritise and Schedule time for self-care activities:** that make you

feel good about yourself, make self-care a priority. Receiving gentle massages, taking warm baths, getting adequate sleep, employing relaxation methods such as deep breathing or meditation, and engaging in interests or pursuits that make you happy and calm can all contribute to this.

- **Connect with others:** Make friends with other pregnant mothers or join pregnancy support agencies to gain a sense of connection and emotional support. It can be beneficial and enjoyable to share concerns, experiences, and suggestions with others who are going through similar transitions

Pre-natal ceremonies:

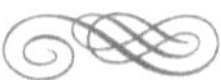

The ancients respected the innate understanding of the synchronicity of human life and its connection the cycle of nature. All the laws and customs they formed were based on nature, with the understanding that when man follows nature all life exists in harmony.

Consequently harmony begets peace and where there is peace there is an understanding of co-existence of all living beings in unity with all living things.

All life is spiritual. Spirit is the air, the breath, the enegry which keeps the body alive. Spirit is the ethereal part of man. The Bible; Genesis 2:7 - Then the LORD God formed a man from dust of the ground and breathed into his nostrils the breath of life, and the man became a living being.

When a person's breath stops the person's body ceases to exist. Upon death the "spirit returns back to God who gave it" Ecclesiastes 12:7 othe excerpts are from Job: 34:14-15 and Psalm: 104: 29-30.

The life of an African is full of ritual ceremonies. Just to make it clear for some who don't realise we all live a ritualistic life, whether by conscious or unconscious design. Rituals exist in eveyy nation, culture and society.

All the calenders of nations like the Chinese or Indian or Gregorian calenders are a rtiual programme for the nations that live by them.

In observation and or celebration of ceremonies like New Year's Day, Valentines Day, Easter, The Jubilee, Workers's Day, Remembrance Sunday, Guy Folks or Christmas Day. All these are rituals with different names for different purposes, like all rituals are.

In an African household, as with all cultures, the arrival of a new baby is an occasion for celebration. The traditional ceremonies start before the baby is born and may continue for up to a year after birth. Various rituals and customs mark this period of time.

Throughout pregnancy, suitable excerpts from the family praise names are poetically recited to evoke happiness and good vibrations, accompanied by

singing, and drumming to appease appeasing divinity. With the aim of producing an auspicious environment for the growth of the child in the womb that is being nurtured by the mother-to-be.

Women are encouraged to avoid going to any places with unsavoury atmospheres like bars and pubs, and even funerals. And to be conscious of the pictures and decor they keep in their homes. Also encouraged to avoid meanering about, because every space they walk into has an energy that affects the the expectant woman and the formation of the soul of their unborn child.

Everything we absorb with our senses; Seeing, Hearing, Smelling, Tasting, and Touching form part of our soul. Even our skin absorbes evnergy through the pores. It is therefore important to choose artmospheres that conntribute positively to our ever evolving soules and in particular for the soul of an un born baby. Giving a positive foundsation upon which their soul is developed.

People are born-again everyday, influenced by experiences, constantly changing and evolving all the time whether consciously or unconsviously for the better or worse depends on how aware an individual is about their thoughts and actions.

At every stage of an African there are rituals. All life is a ritual whether designed with or without the will of the people in every family, society and or nation.

Each ceremony is intended to help sanctify the person, and make them a better and fitter person to enter a particular phase of life. In this instant, a man and woman planning to become pregnant would seek blessings through prayer and cleansing with the help of a Shaman, this would include following a strict diet to detox followed by a nourishing diet for both the father and mother-to-be, cleanse their home where they reside to appease good energy.

In the African culture, ceremonies are performed by the Shaman in the form of rituals and sacrifices. In all the socio-spiritual ceremonies, the women from the village or town's neighbourhood gather in numbers and prepare the embellishments and food before the ceremony.

They are mainly purification in nature and serve two purposes;

The First ceremony is to remove obstacles or ward off evil energy, and to pray for Divine beneficial results. Some of these rituals are social and others are socio-spiritual.

The First ceremony is performed at the end of the third month or the beginning of the fourth month of pregnancy.

In this ritual, before sunrise, the woman takes a shower, and thereafter gets into a steam bath with water flavoured with a mixture of herbs and flowers for cleansing, and the incense is burned toenhance a calming artmosphere.

For example, all parents wish to be blessed with a healthy child, intelligent, diligent, and good-looking. The husband, father-to-be ceremony would give more attention to praying for his wife's conception of good offspring. That the Divine Creator may make his wife, a mother-to-be, fit. So the child is born healthy.

After the child has been conceived, there are two important pre-natal ceremonies performed;

Before the birth of the child. In both rituals the aim is about the well-being of the unborn child, as well as the mother-to-be as the the centre of attention. The father-to-be also takes part in this ritual all under the guidance of the Shaman, because, the rituals are predominantly female-orientated.

The Third part of the ritual, the woman then bathes in water flavoured with a mixture of flower petals believed to adorn her aura with beautiful energy. All this is accompanied by the woman drinking a herbal portion to help her metabolic system stay in balance. This is accompanied by a prayer for the birth of a child.

Beads are significant symbols and codes

Special beads are usually prepared by an elderly woman of the community or the Shaman. The woman wears a beaded necklace and bracelet on the left wrist as a way of protection.

The second aspect of the ceremony is performed between the end of the sixth month of pregnancy. The mother-to-be wears another beaded bracelet on the right wrist.

These bangles are usually dressed by the community elder woman or a Shaman when people live in the city, often these ceremonies are conducted with selected family and perhaps a few trusted friends of the family. And at this stage, it is a women-only ceremony.. Songs of praise and gratitude to the Divine and songs of wellness are sung. Food is served by the family to give thanks to those present in the ceremony.

The last ceremony before childbirth, takes place on the eighth month of pregnancy. With the help of the Shaman and the presence of the village's elderly women. The mother-to-be is massaged with oil-containing oils to relax the muscles of the woman. And some oil is poured on her head and massaged gently to ease her mind and help her keep a relaxed state of mind. Songs of gratitude, love, beauty, and affluence are sung in praise of the Divine for their blessings. Songs depicting heroism if it would be a boy child and nurturing if be a girl child.

People who rigidly follow modern-day lifestyles dismiss all this as superstition without the understanding that whether one is conscious or not, all life is a ritual of ceremonies. The difference is some rituals are ancient well thought out phylosophies that have served humanity in a positive way. Compared to the so-called Western medical fraternity's civilised ways, which totally ignore and ridicule the spiritual aspect of life. All life is spiritual. Only determined by the Medical and pharmaceutical forces of modern-day lifestyles.

People who rigidly follow modern-day lifestyles dismiss all this as superstition without the understanding that whether one is conscious or not, all life is a ritual of ceremonies.

The difference is some rituals are ancient well thought out phylosophies that have served humanity in a positive way which totally ignore and ridicule the spiritual aspect of life.

Health

What is health? This word is always on the tip of our tongue. We've all had direct experience with the agony of being sick, whether it's a slight headache or a long-term condition. Health is an inside job.

So, being in good health refers to a condition of physical, mental, and social well-being in which a person is free of illness, injury, or disease. It is a wide notion that encompasses many facets of overall well-being.

Following a traumatic occurrence, we become aware of how fragile we may be. We realise that our health is exclusively our individual responsibility because the body belongs to the individual, not the government, the health insurance provider, or the nurse or doctor.

We now understand how critical it is to care for our own physical, mental, and spiritual well-being. Your power to influence your overall well-being is solely dependent on your actions and choices.

Health is not merely the absence of disease, but rather the phrase "health" refers to a complete state of physical, mental, and social well-being that extends beyond the absence of disease. Lifestyle choices, environmental impacts, access to healthcare, and socioeconomic factors are only a few of the factors that influence it. Promoting and maintaining good health involves adopting a holistic approach that considers all aspects of well-being.

Physical health: refers to the state of having all of the body's systems, organs, and physiological processes functioning normally. It considers factors like eating well, exercising, getting adequate sleep, and not becoming sick or injured.

Mental health refers to a person's mental, emotional, and psychological well-being. Including aspects such as emotional fortitude, stress tolerance, a strong sense of self-worth, and the absence of mental health concerns.

Social health: A person's social health relates to the quality of their connections, interactions, and social networks. It involves communicating constructively with others, maintaining healthy relationships, friendships, and participating in social activities.

Adopting a comprehensive strategy that considers all aspects of wellness is required to establish and maintain excellent health.

Develop and practice healthy habits, and seek information about the changes in your environment and, how that change affects the food you eat. Food has a significant impact on your well-being, your state of mind, and consequently your mood. All this energy becomes your vibration, if it is negative you then attract people with the same aura into your space, on the contrary, if it is positive you then attract like people.

Physical and spiritual wellness: Surrender to love and to the power of the infinite intellect, which gives us all life. The environment, organisms, and all other living things are all included. Seek counsel from a trusted professional, who is passionate about healing. Having solid connections, leading a balanced lifestyle, and dealing with stress are all important.

Health is not merely the absence of disease. Rather, The phrase "health" refers to a complete state of physical, mental, and social well-being that extends beyond the absence of disease. Numerous factors influence it, including genetics, lifestyle, environment, access to healthcare, and socioeconomic concerns.

Health is an inside job. To develop and maintain excellent health, a comprehensive plan that considers all aspects of life to achieve well-being is required. Holistic health is an inside job and it all begins in mind. Requiring a deliberate and consciously positive perspective of life which results in a balanced lifestyle.

This includes leading a balanced lifestyle, practicing healthy behaviours, seeking regular health care, managing stress, engaging in positive relationships.

It is very important for a woman to detox the clutter from her mind as well as her physical environment before embarking on her pregnancy journey. It's a new phase never lived before. In most ancient cultures, including my African culture, a sacred space has to be prepared both mentally and physically to give the creation of this sacred manifestation the best platform.

Everything in life co-exists in tandem with its polar opposite. To live a life of pure pleasure, freedom, harmony, and love with nature and all people on the earth, you must keep your spirit, body, and mind in balance.

Be mindful and conscious of your thoughts because they form your emotions and consequently you create your experiences.

Chapter 2: Detox Your Body and Mind

Preparing your mind, emotions **and body for a healthy pregnancy**

This preparation includes focusing on your overall well-being and making good lifestyle choices.While the term "detox" can have different interpretations, here are some basic tips to keep a healthy mind and body before pregnancy:

Eat a well balanced diet: Rich in whole foods such as fruits, vegetables, whole grains, lean meats, and healthy fats. Limit your intake of processed foods with artificial additives, sugar, and unnatural ingredients. Stay well-hydrated by drinking an adequate amount of water as per your body requirement.

Engage in regular physical activity: Regularly engage in moderate exercise into your routine, such as walking, swimming, yoga, or prenatal fitness classes. Consult with your healthcare provider to determine appropriate exercise recommendations for your individual circumstances.

Explore and experiment stress-reduction techniques: such as deep breathing exercises, meditation, yoga, or mindfulness activities. You can reduce stress by engaging in uplifting activities, enjoy time in nature, and maintaining a healthy work-life balance can also help reduce stress.

Get sufficient sleep: Prioritise getting enough sleep to improve and support your overall well-being. restful sleep depends on each individual.

So, create a sleep-friendly environment and establish a consistent sleep routine that suits you. The number of sleeping hours may vary between seven and eight hours, depending on a person's daytime intellectual and or physical activities.

Minimise exposure to toxins: To accomplish this, reduce your exposure to harmful substances. Avoid smoking, drinking alcohol, and using recreational drugs. Lessen your exposure to environmental pollutants such as pesticides, common household cleaners, and some cosmetics. Discuss any specific concerns you have with your healthcare provider.

Seek emotional support: Surround yourself with a network of loving family members, close friends, or a trained therapist. Address any emotional or psychological issues, and seek treatment or counselling if necessary.

Prioritise self-care: Make rest and wellbeing a high priority. Bathing, hobbies, finding creative outlets, or engaging in delightful activities that make you happy and serene can all contribute to this.

Schedule preconception check-ups: Check in with your healthcare provider for preconception check-ups to ensure you are up to date on screenings. Make pre-conception appointments. Discuss any pre-existing health conditions, medications, or concerns related to your pregnancy plans.

Learn about pregnancy: Educate yourself and learn about childbirth, and newborn care. Prenatal workshops or classes can help you learn about pregnancy health problems including nutrition and exercise.

Consultations: Remember, it's always important to consult with your healthcare provider before making any significant changes to your lifestyle or starting any new practices. They can provide personalised advice based on your specific health needs and circumstances.

Women can eat to Prevent Pregnancy Diabetes

This book should be read by every woman who desires to have a baby. Who is expecting to become a mother, and mothers who are seeking for natural ways to avoid, treat, or aid in the recovery of one of the most ferocious diseases in the world, Diabetes. One of the fastest growing diseases in the world.

Diabetes is a greek word meaning; one who regularly urinates.

Our way of life, particularly in large cities where many people eat little naturally grown food straight from "Mother Earth," preferring to buy pre-packaged and processed meals, is clearly at the foundation of this grave threat to humanity.

The digestion process of foods containing; carbohydrates, protein, minerals and vitamins:

The digestion process involves breaking down different types of food components to release their nutrients for absorption into the body.

Consider how diets high in minerals, vitamins, carbohydrates, and protein digest:

Carbohydrates:

- Digestion starts at the tip of your fork or your spoon, or perhaps the bite size at the tips of your fingers if you eat suing your hands. Then goes to your mouth, where the enzyme amylase in saliva begins to break down complex carbohydrates into simpler sugars.

• In the stomach, carbohydrates face minimal digestion as the acidic environment halts the action of amylase.

• The majority of carbohydrate digestion occurs in the small intestine.

• Pancreatic amylase and enzymes produced by the small intestine break down complex carbohydrates into glucose, fructose, and galactose.

Protein:

• Protein digestion begins in the stomach, where the enzyme pepsin breaks down proteins into smaller polypeptides.

• Pancreatic enzymes known as proteases further break down polypeptides into amino acids in the small intestine.

These smaller sugar molecules are then transported into the bloodstream to supply energy to the cells.

Minerals:

• Minerals can be absorbed variably depending on other dietary circumstances, regardless of the fact that they are not chemically broken down during digestion.

• Minerals enter the bloodstream via the intestinal lining of the small intestine.

• A variety of factors, including the availability of other nutrients or specific compounds in meals, might influence mineral absorption.

Vitamins:

• Different vitamins digest in different ways depending on the type. While certain vitamins are easily absorbed, others require specific enzymes or processes to be absorbed.

• Dietary lipids are required for the absorption of fat-soluble vitamins (A, D, E, and K). They are absorbed lipids in the small intestine and transported through the lymphatic system.

• Water-soluble vitamins (such as vitamin C and B vitamins) are absorbed directly into the bloodstream and promptly in the small intestine.

Furthermore, it is important to note that, while some nutrients, such as fibre, are necessary for digestion, they are not digested and pass through the body undigested.

Some examples of food containing dietary fibre
Whole Grains:

• Oats
• Brown rice
• Quinoa
• Whole wheat
• Barley
• Bulgur
• Buckwheat

Fruits:

- Apples
- Pears
- Avocado
- Oranges
- Bananas
- Prunes
- Kiwi
- Berries: Raspberries, Strawberries, Blueberries or Bilberries.

Vegetables:

- Artichokes
- Broccoli
- Brussels sprouts,
- Carrots
- Peas
- Spinach
- Sweet potatoes.

Nuts and Seeds:

- Almonds
- Chia seeds
- Flaxseeds
- Pistachios
- Walnuts
- Sunflower seeds.

Legumes:

- Lentils. Chickpeas. Kidney beans. Black beans. Navy beans. Pinto beans. Split peas.

Whole Grains:

• Oats. Brown rice. Quinoa. Whole wheat. Barley. Bulgur. Buckwheat

Bran Cereals:

• Wheat bran. Oat bran. Rice bran

The pancreas' role in food digestion:
The pancreas is a glandular organ located in the abdominal cavity, behind the stomach. It plays an important role in the digestive system by producing enzymes and hormones that aid in the breakdown of food and the absorption nutrients.

The pancreas has two fundamental **functions:**
Exocrine Function: Exocrine cells manufacture and secrete digestive enzymes and make up the majority of the pancreas. Amylase, lipase, and proteases are digestive enzymes that are released into the small intestine to break down proteins, carbohydrates, and lipids into smaller molecules that the body may absorb more easily. This technique aids in the digestion and absorption of nutrients.

• Endocrine Function: Scattered throughout the pancreas are five types of clusters of cells called islets of Langerhans. These islets contain five types of specialised cells that produce and release hormones directly into the bloodstream. The pancreas contains 500 endocrine cells.

• The Alpha cell cluster is the only clump of Langerhans islets. The Alpha cells cluster breaks down glycogen, a substance generated in bodily tissues as a repository for carbs that are converted to glucose in the liver.

• The Delta cells are another cluster that produces the pituitary gland hormones; somatostatin which controls hormone release, gastrointestinal activity, and cell reproduction. And ghrelin is a hormone produced and released by the stomach. It alerts your brain that your stomach is empty and that it is time to eat, which controls the endocrine system.

• Hormones send signals to organs, skin, muscles, and other tissues via blood. These signals tell your body what to do—or stop doing—and when The endocrine system is a looping reaction of hormones released by internal glands of the body directly into the Blood Circulatory system, which includes the heart, the blood arteries blood itself. The pancreas also secretes the delta cell cluster.

• The pancreas primarily produces the hormones insulin and glucagon to regulate blood sugar levels. Glucagon raises blood sugar by pushing the liver's stored glucose to be released, whereas insulin lowers blood sugar by allowing glucose uptake into cells.

In summary, digestive enzymes are produced by the pancreas' exocrine cells and are essential for breaking down food and boosting nutrient absorption in the small intestine. Endocrine cells in the pancreas secrete hormones that regulate blood sugar levels, making them crucial to metabolism as a whole.

What causes diabetes

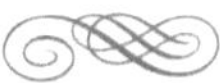

Mitochondrial Dysfunction and the Diseases it causes

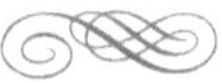

Mitochondrial dysfunction refers to impaired or disrupted functioning of the mitochondria, which are the energy-producing organised structures within a cell. Mitochondria are responsible for generating adenosine triphosphate (ATP), the cell's primary energy unit. When mitochondrial activity is reduced, it can cause various diseases and health conditions.

The following are some illnesses associated with mitochondrial dysfunction:

- Mitochondrial diseases: These hereditary disorders have a direct impact on mitochondrial function. They may have an effect on the nervous system, muscles, heart, liver, and kidneys, among other organs.

Examples of mitochondrial diseases include mitochondrial encephalopathy, lactic acidosis, and stroke-like episodes (MELAS), Leigh syndrome, and mitochondrial myopathy.

- Neurodegenerative diseases: Many neurodegenerative illnesses, including Alzheimer's, Parkinson's, Huntington's, and amyotrophic lateral sclerosis (ALS), are known to be influenced by mitochondrial dysfunction.

- increased oxidative stress, and neural malfunction, all of which can lead to the progression of various illnesses.

• Metabolic disorders: Mitochondrial dysfunction can disrupt normal metabolic functions and create a variety of issues. For example, difficulties with mitochondrial activity may make it difficult to break down fatty acids, resulting in illnesses such as fatty acid oxidation disorders. Other metabolic diseases associated to mitochondrial dysfunction include diabetes, obesity, and insulin resistance.

- Cardiovascular diseases: Heart failure, ischemic heart disease, and cardiomyopathy are just a few of the conditions that mitochondrial dysfunction can aggravate. Inadequate ATP generation and severe oxidative stress inside cardiac cells might impair the heart's ability to function efficiently.

ATP is an abbreviation for adenosine triphosphate, which is the primary molecule in cells for storing and transferring energy. ATP is sometimes referred to as the cell's energy - currency. People often say that ATP is the cell's energy-currency exchange, which is like putting money in a bank. Because, similarly to banking, ATP can be used to store energy for future chemical reactions or be withdrawn to use for chemical reactions when the cell needs energy.

- Age-related diseases: It is believed that mitochondrial dysfunction plays a role in ageing and age-related diseases. Increased oxidative damage and lower energy output can arise from age-related mitochondrial malfunction.

This could exacerbate age-related disorders such sarcopenia (muscle wasting), frailty, and cognitive decline. Mitochondrial malfunction can manifest itself in a variety of ways depending on the tissues and organs involved. Reduced ATP synthesis, increased oxidative stress, decreased cellular respiration, and changes in mitochondrial DNA are all prevalent symptoms.

To identify and treat mitochondrial dysfunction and related illnesses, a multidisciplinary strategy comprising medical geneticists, neurologists, cardiologists, and other experts is routinely used. Treatment options include supportive care, symptom-management medications, and targeted therapy aiming at increasing mitochondrial activity.

There are two Types of Diabetes;

Type 1 diabetes, which affects those who do not produce insulin, is one of two forms of diabetes.Type 2 diabetes, which affects insulin-resistant people. A condition in which the cells of the body are unable to efficiently use the blood sugar glucose to produce enough energy. As a result of insulin resistance in cells. As a result, blood pressure rises excessively.

Type 1 and Type 2 Diabetes can cause severe health complications.

Diabetes type 1 and Diabetes type 2, both pose substantial health hazards. According to medical experts, Type 1 Diabetes cannot be reversed since the pancreas is targeted by a weakened immune system. Insulin-producing cells are being harmed. As a result, the cells' insulin secretion ceases. Consequently, blood pressure becomes too high. Fortunately, Type 2 Diabetes is reversible since cells can still create insulin despite the imbalance in the body's system.

Chapter 3: Facts About Insulin

What exacly is Insulin?

1. Insulin is a hormone made by your pancreas. And the pancreas is a gland organ that lives under your left rib behind your stomach. Its main function is to digest and turn the food you eat into nutrients that feed the cells in your body.

1. Insulin is a hormone that regulates and lowers your blood sugar levels by allowing glucose to enter your cells.

1. Insulin, which also works as a storage hormone by storing sugar in the muscles and liver, and produces visceral fat.

1. Hormones are communication agents that are created by your glands and circulate in your blood.

1. As a result, insulin and the pancreas are designed to control your blood glucose, which is a key source of energy for living organisms and a component of many different types of carbohydrates in your body.

1. Insulin delivers glucose from the blood and into the cells. At this point, the pancreas is now in charge of releasing digestive enzymes into the small intestine's first portion.

1. After food enters the first segment of the small intestine,

where it reacts with stomach acid and a greenish-brown alkaline fluid that assists digestion. The liver excretes greenish-brown alkaline fluid, which is kept in the gall bladder, which is located beneath the liver in the upper right corner of the stomach.

1. The body, like the subconscious mind, has a responsive circulatory system that runs in a loop. Because insulin is in charge of removing surplus sugar from your blood, the circulatory system ordinarily activates the insulin hormone to remove it.

1. Furthermore, any excess carbohydrates are broken down into sugar, which insulin then converts into fat because its primary function is to produce the hormone that creates visceral fat.

1. Your body stores two types of fat: visceral fat and subcutaneous fat, which is found directly beneath your skin. The fat that underneath your arms and legs may have.

1. On the other hand, Visceral fat is body fat stored within your abdominal chamber as well as the area surrounding your liver, pancreas, and intestines.

1. Carrying and storing a lot of visceral fat is known to be linked to insulin resistance, which can lead to conditions like type 2 diabetes, leaky gut, heart disease, colorectal cancer, Alzheimer's, and glucose intolerance, a condition caused by high blood sugar levels.

1. Your body contains about 1.5 gallon / 5.7 litres of blood. And according to medical research, the average person consumes about 30 teaspoons, which is about 7 grams of sugar every per day.

What exactly is Food ?

Food refers to any substance consumed by living beings that gives nourishment and fosters our growth, development, and overall well-being. It is frequently consumed by both animals and humans in order to obtain important nutrients, energy, and a variety of compounds required for physiological activities.

Food comes in a wide variety of shapes and forms including plants, animals, and other sources. It can be processed, preserved, or cooked in a variety of ways to increase its flavour, texture, and nutritional value. It can be consumed raw or cooked.

Food's primary purpose is to provide essential nutrients, like, water, carbohydrates, proteins, fats, vitamins and minerals. These nutrients are necessary for supporting development and repair, maintaining overall health, and carrying out typical bodily functions and sustaining overall health.

Food is also essential in cultural, social, and emotional settings. It is often associated with traditions, celebrations, and social gatherings. individual tastes and cultural variances in culinary and nutritional practises can have a significant impact on food choices.

Taste, aroma, and texture are sensory aspects of food that affect our eating experience in addition to its nutritional and cultural components.

Overall, food is an essential aspect of human life and existence, it provides us with sustenance, joy, and the opportunity to eat, be nourished and enjoy.

The food you eat shapes your body

The food you eat has a substantial impact on your body through a range of biological processes. Here's an overview of how the food you eat affects the shape of your body:

• **Digestion:** Digestion begins at the tip of your mouth, where saliva and food meet and the meal is crushed into tiny particles. It subsequently travels to the stomach, where it is further degraded by stomach acids and enzymes. After leaving the stomach, where they have only partially digested the meal, nutrients are transported into the bloodstream via the small intestine.

• **Nutrient Absorption:** Nutrients from food are absorbed into the bloodstream in the small intestine. These nutrients include carbohydrates, proteins, fats, vitamins, minerals, and water. The body uses these nutrients for a variety of tasks, including energy production, tissue growth and repair, organ function support, and overall health maintenance.

• **Energy Balance:** The body requires a certain number of calories (or energy) to perform its daily functions. Food energy is used for body processes such as breathing, digestion, movement, and temperature regulation.

• If you consume more calories than your body requires, the excess energy is stored as fat, resulting in weight gain and changes in your body's shape.

- **Body Composition and Macronutrients:** The three macronutrients, carbohydrates, proteins, and fats, are crucial in deciding how your body will look.

- Proteins are required for the formation and repair of tissues, particularly muscles. Eating enough protein, which promotes muscle growth and maintenance, can help you achieve a leaner and more toned body shape.

- **Carbohydrates;** when consumed in excess, can affect body weight and provide energy for physical activities. Fats, when consumed in moderation and from healthy sources, aid in the production of hormones, the insulation of the body, and the preservation of organs.

- **Metabolism;** Individual metabolism and inheritance can influence how the body metabolises and stores food. Because of their quicker or slower metabolic rates, some people may burn calories more quickly and effectively than others.

- **Genetics:** can influence both the distribution of fat accumulation and body shape. It's important to remember, however, that lifestyle factors like nutrition and exercise, as well as heredity, only account for a small amount of how the body develops.

To ensure a healthy body shape and composition, it is critical to eat a balanced and nutritious diet, exercise regularly, and consider factors such as portion sizes and overall calorie intake.

You can keep a body full of energy that will help you live a happy and active life, by choosing a healthy lifestxyle supported by natural food that suits your metabolism, be it a carnivore, omnivore, or vegetarian diet coupled with frequent exercise for strength and flexebility and prayer and meditaion for calm and a piece of mind.

Thoughts have a direct impact on the decisions you make. Thoughts are matter which influence your choices and actions. less natural diet can cause obesity and malnutrition in you, as well as set the stage for your unborn child's IQ and physical height.

Consuming an excessive amount of fast food, packaged foods, and store-bought foods when pregnant may have detrimental consequences on both the mother's and the growing baby's health.

Malnutrition; is one of the potential hazards. Processed and fast food can lead to obesity and malnutrition in a variety of ways.

- **Increased Portion Sizes:** Fast food and processed food portions tend to be larger than recommended serving sizes. Consuming large portion sizes regularly can lead to calorie excess and weight gain. Over time, the excess calories can contribute to obesity.

- **Impact on Satiety and Food Choices:** Processed foods and fast food are often low in fibre and protein, which are important for promoting satiety and keeping us feeling full. These foods are typically high in calories but low in volume, making it easier to over consume without feeling satisfied.

Understanding How Store-Bought Processed Food and Fast Food Contribute to Malnutrition:

Ingredients in fast foods **can contribute to weight gain and obesity.**

Nutrient Density Deficit: Fast food and processed foods can be high in calories but low in key nutrients. They may be supplemented with synthetic analogues, although they are frequently treated to eliminate essential components. This means that, while they provide energy in the form of calories, they are lacking in the vitamins, minerals, and fibre required for optimal health.

Despite consuming an excessive amount of calories, eating these meals on a regular basis may result in vitamin deficiency and malnutrition.

Fast food and processed foods are high in unhealthy components such as trans fats, saturated fats, added sugars, refined carbohydrates, and an excessive quantity of sodium. These chemicals may play a role in weight gain and obesity.

Refined carbohydrates and added sugars; can all lead to increased fat storage, insulin resistance, and blood sugar irregularities. Unhealthy fats increase the risk of heart disease and weight gain. Excessive salt consumption may cause high blood pressure and water retention.

Highly Addictive and Palatable: Processed foods and fast food are frequently designed to be incredibly tasty by combining salt, sugar, and unhealthy fats in combinations that stimulate the brain to feel good. This can lead to overeating and a lack of self-control when it comes to food. The addictive properties of certain foods may also induce excessive calorie intake and weight growth, which can lead to obesity.

Larger portions: The portions of fast food and processed foods are usually larger than recommended serving sizes. Eating large servings on a regular basis may result in calorie excess and weight gain. Obesity may develop as a result of the additional calories.

Impact on Food Choices and Satiety: Fast food and processed foods usually lack the fibre and protein we need to stay satiated and full. These foods are usually low in volume but high in calories, making it easier to take more than you need before feeling satisfied.

The growing availability and convenience of processed meals and fast food may result in an imbalanced and nutritionally insufficient diet.

While regular consumption of fast food or processed foods can contribute to obesity and malnutrition, these options are essentially unhealthy and should be avoided.

To guarantee adequate nutrient intake and, a balanced diet of whole, unprocessed foods should be prioritised to maintain a healthy weight.

As a result, the body is out of balance. Sluggishness is a warning sign that

your body is under stress as a result of eating artificially sweetened meals.

To help normalise and maintain a healthy, balanced glucose and sugar level. When you purchasing food, especially pre-packaged foods from supermarkets, it is best to read the labels.

Too much sugar in your system slows you down.

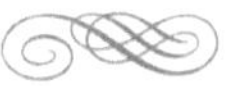

As a result, the body is out of balance. Lethargy is a warning sign that your body is under stress as a result of eating artificially sweetened meals.

To help normalise and maintain a healthy, balanced glucose, sugar level. Check, when purchasing food, especially pre-packaged foods from supermarkets, it is best to read the labels. Specifically, the amount of sugar, carbs, and fat contained in the product.

It is advisable to become acquainted with the numerous names for sugar. Fortunately, the majority of us have easy internet connection.

It is advisable to become acquainted with the numerous names for sugar.

As a result, even if you come across a word that you are unable to both pronounce and understand. You can search up its meaning right away.

Sugar is the common term for soluble carbohydrates with a sweet taste. The names of processed sugars usually end with "ose."

Sugar has several different names:

Types of Carbohydrates;

1. Monosaccharides:
2. Disaccharides
3. Oligosaccharides and
4. Polysaccharides

Examples of Monosaccharides:

1. Glucose

1. Fructose
2. Galactose sometimes abbreviated as Gal

3. Dextrose

1. Levulose

Examples of Disaccharides:

1. Sucrose
2. Lactose
3. Maltose
4. Maltobiose

Simple Sugar

1. Honey
2. Sugar cane
3. Sugar Beet

Refiners Syrup
Refiners Syrup, is actually sugar.

1. Rice Syrup
2. Corn Syrup

Examples of Polysaccharides are;

1. Cellulose
2. Starch
3. Chitin

Examples of Disaccharides:

1. Sucrose
2. Lactose

Brown Rice Malt Syrup.1

Four Types of Carbohydrates

Carbohydrates are another name for starch, a form of glucose found in green plants that is the most common source of energy in human meals. Depending on the consistency desired, more water may be added.

Carbohydrates are another name for starch, a form of glucose found in green plants that is the most common source of energy in human meals.

A little more extra water allows for a lengthier simmering procedure at a little higher temperature to achieve a thicker texture for the syrup.

The syrup is then condensed in a vacuum evaporator to maintain the colour, like in pre-packaged fruit juices.

Sucrose is also called granulated, regular or table sugar

Caution: To make sucrose, most starches have 50% fructose and 50% glucose.

Sucrose is another name for saccharose. It is pure sugar that has been refined from green plants and prepared for human consumption.

Sucrose is a form of sugar that is commonly used in hospitality settings such as hotels, taverns, and restaurants. and are largely used in households around the world.

Glucose is the most common monosaccharide among all carbohydrates.

Monosaccharide is the Greek term for sugar; monos means only one and saccharide signifies sugar. When consuming high amounts of processed sugar, it is prudent to exercise caution.

It is possible to eliminate all forms of processed sugar from your diet. You can; all you have to do is do it for free and change your mind! Syrup is a frequent name for monosaccharides.

Monosaccharide are Commonly Known as Syrup

Syrup, which denotes a sweet solution, is primarily used and preferred by bakers. They primarily use it in cakes and donuts to retain moisture for a fresh flavour.

It is possible to eliminate all forms of processed sugar from your diet. You can; all you have to do is do it for free and change your mind! Syrup is a frequent name for monosaccharides.

Monosaccharides are Commonly Known as Syrup

Syrup, which denotes a sweet solution, is primarily used and preferred by bakers. They primarily use it in cakes and donuts to retain moisture for a fresh flavour.

Plain Simple Sugar is Sweeter than Table Sugar

Simple sugars are sweet-flavoured soluble carbohydrates. It is often known as syrup and is used in jams and jellies. Simple syrup, often known as simple sugar, is a fructose and glucose mixture. This mixture produces a liquid sweetener that is sweeter than table sugar.

Monosaccharide is the Greek term for sugar; monos means only one and saccharide signifies sugar. When consuming high amounts of processed sugar, it is prudent to exercise caution. It is possible to eliminate all forms of processed sugar from your diet. You can; all you have to do is do it for free and change your mind! Syrup is a frequent name for monosaccharides.

Monosaccharides are also the building blocks of Polysaccharides.

Polysaccharides contain several different forms of starch, they are also known as carbs. Rice, potatoes, maize, wheat, bread, cakes, cookies, and doughnuts all include different types of polysaccharides that are stored as starch, as do alcoholic beverages such as cocktails.

Polysaccharides are also known as starch or carbs.

Polysaccharides serve numerous functions. Some people's bodies have energy reserves. Others send cellular messages across the body.

Alcohol is made from natural starch and sugar.

Many alcoholic beverages contain various levels of sugar depending on how they are fermented and distilled. Alcohol is made from natural starch and sugar. Many alcoholic beverages contain various levels of sugar depending on how they are fermented and distilled.

Malted grains' syrup is also used in a variety of beverages including alcoholic drinks like: Bear and Whiskey.

Alcohol is made from natural starch and sugar.

Many alcoholic beverages contain various levels of sugar depending on how they are fermented and distilled.

During the fermentation process, enzymes deconstruct into glucose, resulting in the creation of glucose molecules. Although polysaccharides are difficult to digest, they provide nutritional fibre. As a result, these enzymes aid digestion depending on the degree of fermentation.

Sugar has a plethora of names since it is derived from a wide range of plants and processed in a variety of methods depending on its intended use. Malt syrup, for example, is made from cereal grains.

Enzymes produced by malting grains are required for the conversion

of starches in grains to sugar. In stage one of the three-step malting process, the grains are steeped in water for germination. The seeds' germination is halted in stage two. Heat is employed to dry the grains in the third stage.

The malting process converts barley or other cereal grains into malt, which is used in brewing. Because these sugars are already present in the grain used to manufacture beer or whisky, they have not been transformed into starch.

Starchy cereals such as wheat and barley are converted into sugar during the traditional malting process. Pressing the plant juice yields a significant amount of sugar. Following then, the juice is dried up.

Inverted sugar syrup can be created, without the assistance of **acids or enzymes.**

Fruit juice that has evaporated into the air crystallises and is generally known as inverted sugar or concentrated juice, such as grape juice.

Granulated sugar and water in a 2:1 ratio are the only two ingredients required to manufacture it.

Depending on the consistency desired, more water may be added.

A little more extra water allows for a lengthier simmering procedure at a little higher temperature to achieve a thicker texture for the syrup.

The syrup is then condensed in a vacuum evaporator to maintain the colour, like in pre-packaged fruit juices Simple sugars like fructose, glucose, and sucrose contribute in the fermentation process. Thus, fermentation is achievable with any invert sugar formulation.

Inverted sugar syrup can be made by heating table sugar dissolved in water.

Sugar inversion can be accomplished fast by mixing sugar with citric acid, cream of tartar, or lemon juice. The mixture, which has a weight-to-water content ratio of 1000:1, is supposed to prevent crystallisation.

Cinnamon has a citric acid content of 5% by weight. As a result, when lemon is used for sugar inversion, the ratio changes from 1000:1 to 50:1. When the sugar and lemon mixture is heated at 114o C and added to another food without tasting sour, the mixture inversion prevents crystallisation.

Added Sugars vs. Free Sugars

Free sugar is low in nutrients. Since our childhood, most of us have been aware of the health risks connected with drinking sweetened beverages. Consuming sugar causes tooth decay and weight gain, which can lead to obesity, diabetes, and heart disease. This is because free sugar, also known as refined sugar, has no nutritious value because it is entirely composed of calories.

Sugar, whether free or refined, is devoid of minerals, fibre, and protein. Sugar induces a "bliss point" in the brain system of the person who consumes it, making it just as addictive as cocaine

Gustav Theodore Fechner, a scientist, philosopher, and experimentalist, was born in Leipzig, an industrial city in East Central Germany. He concentrated his studies on physical stimuli and how they connect to the nature or aspects of awareness in the mind.

He released a book named "Elements of Psychophysics," also known as "Elements of Psychophysics. "

As a result, he is regarded as the father of psychophysics, the study of stimuli, perceptions, and sensations. His efforts were focused on developing a way for connecting matter and the mind.

Fechner sought to connect the externally apparent world to an individual's experience and perception of it. the "Bliss Point" in the brain brought on by a diet heavy in fat, salt, and sugar.

Howard Moskowitz, an American market researcher and psychophycisist, discovered the "Bliss Point" in the 1990s.

The "Bliss Point" is a state of extreme pleasure that happens in the human brain after consuming a combination of sugar, salt, and fat.

Prepackaged sauces are highly processed, containing additional salt, sugar, and fat.

Examine the containers' components and do the arithmetic to see how much your family would consume monthly or even annually.

Making these sauces at home is really simple, and it allows you to use fresh, organic products that will not only taste your cuisine to your liking, and will also boost the nutritional value of your meals.

Chapter 4: Sweeteners From Nature

Low Processed Sweeteners From Trees, Plant Fruits or Insects
Honey is sweet due to its high concentration of glucose and fructose, two sugars derived from the previously mentioned monosaccharides known as simple sugars. We've all heard about it, honey. It is made by honey bees.

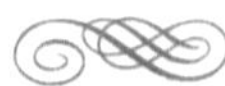

Plants Insects and trees' juice are widely used to create sugar.

Because flowers rely on bee pollination, the honey is then stored to feed bee colonies that pollinate the flowers.

Bees are essential for flowers to exist and give us with beauty for our eyes to feast on. There is also aroma to pleasure our senses and savour the sweetness of life. Bee pollination is also critical to fruit production.

To make honey, bees collect and purify nectar secreted by flowers and plants.

The honey is then stored in honeycomb hives made of wax.

Honey is obtained either from domestic bee hives or from wild bee colonies. The honey is then stored in honeycomb hives made of wax.

Honey is obtained either from domestic bee hives or from wild bee colonies.

Honey should never be heated or cooked. According to Ayurveda, heating or cooking with honey changes its natural structure and releases harmful compounds that stick to the mucous membrane of the digestive tract.

Honey is best ingested in its natural state because it is high in vitamins C, D, E, K, and B-Complex. Aside from the numerous other natural benefits, honey contains enzymes, minerals, amino acids, beta-carotene, essential oils, and antioxidants, to mention a few. We are thankful for bees. They should be treated with love and respect for future generations.

Palms are the most extensively grown trees on the planet and come in a wide range of variations.

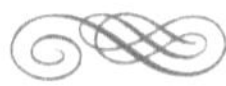

Palm sweeteners are made from many sorts of palm trees.

Because palm sugar is made from a variety of palm trees, it is identified by the palm tree from which it is gathered. The juice thickens into a saccharide compound that can be sold as palm syrup after further heating.

Coconut sugar crystallises over time, at which point it is offered as bricks or cakes. Coconut palm sugar has a particular flavour depending on where it is manufactured. Honey's colour can range from golden yellow to chestnut brown, depending on how it is stored.

Fluid of Natural Plant-Based Sugars

Cane sugar is a plant native to India and Africa.

- Sugarcane is refined into sugar. Sugarcane is converted into a syrupy liquid after processing. This thick consistency is then utilised to make various sweeteners.

Raw sugar, also known as jaggery, brown sugar, beetroot syrup, and demerara are all sugarcane-derived sweeteners.

• Agave syrup, often known as agave nectar, is derived from the agave plant. The two most well-known agave species are Blue Agave and Agave-Salmiana, Agave syrup, often known as agave nectar, is derived from the agave plant.

• The two most well-known agave species are Blue Agave and Agave-Salmiana, which are native to the Canary Islands in Spain, Italy, and South Africa and thrive mostly in the southern portion of Mexico.

• The agave plant must mature for seven to fourteen years before the syrup can be obtained. To get the juice from the plant's core, the leaves must first be removed.

• The juice from the agave plant is finely condensed after filtering to make syrup. It has a light to dark amber hue and a texture that is frequently thinner than honey.

• Birch syrup is made from birch tree nectar, which is used to flavour soft drinks, ice cream, wine, and beer. Birch syrup is also used to glaze fish and hog dishes.

Sugarcane Nutritional Values

Natural, unprocessed cane sugar is not only delicious but also sweet. Because of its high sugar content and hard texture, it is impossible to consume too much of it. It, like other fruits, is best consumed in moderation because it contains nutritional value:

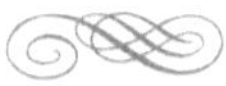

Sugar cane has trace amounts of iron, magnesium, potassium, and phosphorus. Vitamins B1 and B2 are also present, albeit in little quantities. It contains a high concentration of vitamin C.

Be cautious; cane sugar is regularly advertised as a healthier alternative to table sugar. Be wary of processed cane sugar, which contains fructose and glucose, both sucrose-based sugars.

Because of its excessive sweetness, it becomes a sweetener that can drastically impair your health and cause insulin resistance, which can lead to obesity and Type 2 diabetes, among other problems.

Dates Sugar: Sugar made from palm dates. Please keep in mind that date sugar and date palm sugar, often known as wild date palm, are two completely different items. Barley malt syrup is created by extracting sprouting malt syrup from the plant. Breakfast cereals and bread are also made with barley syrup.

Palm tree is native to Mauritius and can also be found in Bangladesh, India, Nepal, and Sri Lanka.

Date Palm Sugar Date palm tree fruit is used to make both wine and jelly. Fresh fruit juice, as well as juice fermented into a hot toddy, can be eaten.

- A Hot Toddy is a beverage that contains an alcoholic beverage such as whisky, as well as spices such as cinnamon, date palm sugar, and/or honey. This beverage is popular in the winter, particularly in England.

- Maple syrup is made from the juice of maple trees. In colder climates such as Canada and the United States, maple trees store starch in their roots and trunks before winter.

- Maple syrup is extracted from trees in the late winter and early spring by boring holes in their trunks and collecting the fluid discharge. During the operation, the fluid is heated to assist as much water evaporate as possible, allowing the condensed syrup to be extracted.

- The Canadian province of Quebec produces the most maple syrup, accounting for 70% of the global supply.

- Panela sugar: is available in two colours of brown; light and dark. It is available in a variety of forms, including liquid, solid blocks, granulated, and crystallised.

- Panela is pure, unrefined whole cane sugar that has not been processed in any way. Panela is extensively available in Central and Latin America. It is manufactured from crushed sugarcane.

• Panela sweetener is also used in the production of vinegar, beer, and wine, as well as canned products, baking, confections, soft drinks, and confections.

Sugar Mascavado

Despite the fact that muscovado is made from cane sugar, the procedure is slightly different. It is made utilising the all-natural method of extracting sugar from sugar cane juice by evaporating water.

• Muscovado is made from a combination of unrefined and refined sugar and has molasses as its principal component, flavour, and colour, giving it a dark brown appearance.

• Despite the fact that it includes minerals, muscovado sugar is just as bad for your health as table sugar. It, along with all other sugars, can cause problems such as obesity, type 2 diabetes, and heart attacks, cavity, to name a few.

Maple syrup is also advertised as a healthier alternative to regular sugar.

It is also a processed sweetener that, when consumed in large quantities, can cause blood sugar swings and insulin resistance.

Polyphenol antioxidants present in unprocessed pure maple juice, on the other hand, can help reduce the risk of heart disease, arthritis, and inflammation.

It improves digestion and supplies zinc and magnesium to the immune system when consumed in moderation. The maple leaf.

Maple trees

Maple trees appear in a variety of striking sizes and colours, especially in the autumn. Trees can be grown using one of two methods: seeds or tree cuttings.

Mid-summer or mid-autumn are the optimal periods to plant maple trees from cuttings of young maple trees. After cutting the tip of the young trees, remove the leaves from the lower half of the stem to successfully reproduce roots from stem cuttings.

Rooting hormones can help roots form faster and with higher quality roots. Maple trees, especially in the autumn, enhance the beauty of the landscape.

Birch trees generate clear, slightly sweet, and fresh water.

The water is slightly thicker than water and has a lovely, cooling flavour.

A slightly sweet and woody flavour. Birch beer comes in a variety of flavours.

Birch sap is a key ingredient in all of them. Despite the fact that some birch beers are carbonated non-alcoholic soft drinks. Others are created using alcohol through a fermentation process that converts birch sap into alcohol. Baking yeast is occasionally used in the production process for fermentation.

Silver Birch Trees

Iron, calcium, magnesium, manganese, potassium, and phosphorus are all minerals contained in silver birch sap that help with bone growth and preservation. Keep in mind that certain birch water brands contain refined birch sugar.

Birch sap is used to make products such as mead, an alcoholic beverage prepared from fermented honey and birch water. a couple wines, sugar, and birch syrup.

The optimal time to extract birch water is after autumn and early spring to collect the sweet tasting water before the leaves turn green. so that the water does not taste bitter.

Date palm trees thrive in both subtropical and tropical climates and come in a variety of sizes, shapes, and flavours.

Dates are grown in the Middle East, North Africa, and South Asia. Because of their excellent flavour, they have become native to many subtropical and tropical countries.

Dates, in addition to being deliciously sweet, are a good source of energy. Compared to refined sugar, it is healthier. Especially for people with Type 2 Diabetes. Although dates contain natural sugar, they should be consumed in moderation, as with all other foods.

Plants create vitamins, and dates are high in several of them, including vitamins A, B1, B2, and B3. Thiamine, often known as vitamin B1, aids in the conversion of carbohydrates into glucose, which provides energy to the body.

Riboflavin, often known as vitamin B2, is required for the growth, development, and proper operation of the body's cells. Plants absorb minerals created by the soil and water. Dates are therefore abundant in fibre, energy, and antioxidants.

Chapter 5: Fresh Fruit Versus Fruit Juice

The nutritional difference between fresh fruit and fruit juice
The nutritional difference between drinking freshly squeezed fruit juice and eating fresh fruit in its raw, natural state.

Fruits' nutritional content varies depending on whether they are taken raw, in their natural state, or juiced. Here are some things to consider:

• Consuming whole fruits helps you to receive the fruit's fibre, which is beneficial for digestion, blood sugar regulation, and maintaining a healthy weight. Juicing removes the fibre, decreasing the fibre content of the juice.

• Nutrient Concentration: Juicing concentrates the nutrients in fruits, making them easier for the body to absorb. However, some nutrients, particularly those found in the fruit's skin or pulp, may be lost during the juicing process.

• Juicing might result in juice with a higher concentration of natural sugars than eating the fruit whole. This is because drinking fruit juice helps you to eat more fruit, which may result in increased sugar consumption.

• Both raw and freshly juiced fruits include antioxidants, which aid in the body's defence against cellular damage.

• However, some antioxidants may be destroyed if they are exposed to heat or oxygen during the juicing process. Because of the high fibre content of the fruit, eating it whole may improve satiety and a sense of fullness.

Drinking juice, on the other hand, may leave you feeling less full and eating more calories if not supplemented with other nutritional sources.

• It's important to remember that juicing can be a convenient way to include a variety of fruits and vegetables into your diet, especially if you have difficulties consuming them whole. It is generally recommended to prefer whole fruits and vegetables over liquids to ensure you obtain the full complement of nutrients and dietary fibre.

• Consider adding a variety of fruits and vegetables to your juice to boost its nutritious content. To avoid nutritional loss due to oxidation, consume freshly produced juice immediately or store it properly.

• Finally, pay attention to portion sizes and balance your diet with a variety of nutritious meals to suit your nutritional needs.

What happens when you blend fruit or vegetables into a smoothie?

• Making a smoothie from fruits and vegetables may result in some nutritional loss.

• Oxidation: Fruits and vegetables exposed to oxygen during blending may oxidise, resulting in nutrient loss over time. This is especially true for delicate elements like vitamin C.

Exploring the relationship between thecolour of natural food and the nourishment required by the body?

The key reason that binds the hue of natural food to the nourishment required by the body is the presence of diverse phytochemical, biologically active compounds found in plants antioxidants, and nutrients that give food their attribute colours.

Here are a few examples:

★ Foods in the Colours Purple and Red Anthocyanin is commonly found in foods with brightly coloured red or purple tints, such as berries, grapes, pomegranates, and red cabbage. Anthocyanin antioxidants have been associated to improved cardiovascular health, reduced inflammation, and improved cognitive function.

★ Yellow and orange foods include: Carotenoids, particularly beta-carotene, are abundant in orange and yellow-coloured fruits and vegetables such as oranges, carrots, sweet potatoes, and mangoes. Carotenoids, which are converted into vitamin A in the body, are crucial for keeping excellent vision, boosting the immune system, and enhancing skin health.

★ Green foods include: Chlorophyll is the pigment that gives leafy greens such as spinach, kale, and broccoli its colour, as well as green herbs such as parsley and cilantro. Chlorophyll is a powerful antioxidant that aids in detoxifying and provides essential vitamins and minerals such as folate and vitamin K.

★ Blue or blue-green foods include the following: Phycocyanins and anthocyanins are antioxidants present in foods such as blueberries, spirulina, and seaweed.

The anti-inflammatory and antioxidant properties of these chemicals may improve brain function, reduce the risk of chronic illnesses, and improve overall well-being.

★ White or brown foods include the following: These foods may not be brightly coloured, but they are high in nutrients. Sulphur molecules in garlic and onions, for example, support the immune system and heart health. Whole grains, such as brown rice and quinoa, include fibre, B vitamins, and minerals.

How does the food you eat alter the shape of your body?

The food you eat has a substantial impact on your body through a range of biological processes. The following is an outline of how nutrition affects and determines your body shape:

Digestion begins in the mouth, where food is chewed and mixed with saliva to break it down into smaller pieces. It subsequently travels to the stomach, where it is further degraded by stomach acids and enzymes.

After leaving the stomach, where they have only partially digested the meal, nutrients are transported into the bloodstream via the small intestine.

Nutrients Absorption

Nutrients from food are absorbed and delivered to the bloodstream in the small intestine. Among these nutrients are carbohydrates, proteins, fats, vitamins, minerals, and water. The body makes use of these nutrients for various processes, including the creation of energy, the formation and repair of tissues, the support of organ function, and the preservation of overall health.

• The body uses these nutrients for a variety of tasks, including energy production, tissue growth and repair, organ function support, and general health maintenance.

• **Energy Balance:** To perform its daily functions, the body requires a certain number of calories (or energy). Food energy is utilised to power biological activities such as breathing, digestion, movement, and temperature regulation. If you consume more calories than your body requires, the excess energy is stored as fat, resulting in weight gain and changes to your body's shape.

Carbohydrates, when consumed in excess, can have an effect on body weight and provide energy for physical activities. Fats help to generate hormones, insulate the body, and preserve organs when consumed in moderation and from healthy sources.

Individual differences in metabolism and inheritance can influence how the body metabolises and stores food.

Genetics can influence both the location of fat accumulation and the form of the body. It's important to remember, however, that lifestyle decisions like eating and exercise, as well as genes, only account for a small amount of how the body is shaped.

Maintaining a healthy body shape and composition requires a balanced and nutritious diet, frequent physical activity, and consideration of factors such as portion sizes and overall calorie intake.

The potential health repercussions of genetically modified foods (GM foods) have been a matter of debate. Here are some of the issues that have been raised:

• **Allergic reactions:** When genes from one organism are introduced into another, new proteins may be created. These new proteins may trigger allergy reactions in those who are sensitive to them.

• Toxicology: There is concern that genetic changes may result in the production of toxins or other hazardous elements in GM foods. Strict safety evaluations are carried out to ensure that GM foods are not more dangerous than their non-GM counterparts.

• Antibiotic resistance: Antibiotic resistance genes are utilised as markers in numerous genetic engineering methods. Eating GM crops containing these genes raises concerns that bacterial antibiotic resistance will rise.

Several regulatory agencies, however, have demanded that these identifiers be deleted from GM crops used in food.

• The long-term repercussions are unknown: Some argue that because genetic modification technology is still in its early stages, it is unclear how consuming genetically modified crops may effect our health in the long run. Regulatory organisations and long-term studies are still monitoring the safety of GM foods.

• It is important to remember that the scientific community as a whole, including the World Health Organisation (WHO), the National Academy of Sciences, and the European Food Safety Authority, agrees that currently available genetically modified foods are safe to eat.

If the claims made by these organisations is true, why is there such a high increase in the number of chronic diseases in the world. And why do they even have to modify food. You may ask?

• These foods are reported to go through extensive testing and review before being approved for commercialisation. Regulatory groups in several countries have set guidelines and methods to assess the safety of GM foods and ensure they meet predetermined requirements.

An increase in illnesses has presented a threat to humanity since World War You may be wondering what is causing pandemics to spread so swiftly over the planet.

Since World War I, humanity has faced a number of ailments and health problems. Here are a few well-known illnesses:

• Pandemic influenza: The 1918 Spanish Flu outbreak killed millions of people worldwide. Later influenza pandemics, such as the Asian Flu (1957), Hong Kong Flu (1968), and H1N1 Swine Flu (2009), posed major health hazards.

• HIV/AIDS: Since its inception in the 1980s, the HIV/AIDS epidemic has affected millions of individuals worldwide.

It is a viral infection that weakens the immune system and makes people more susceptible to illnesses and infections.

• Cancer: is a severe global health problem characterised by the unregulated development of abnormal cells. Cancers with high mortality rates include lung, breast, colorectal, and prostate cancer.

• Cardiovascular Diseases: Heart disease and stroke are now among the leading causes of death worldwide. Sedentary lifestyles, poor diet, smoking, and high blood pressure are all contributing to an increase in heart disease.

• Type 2 Diabetes which is commonly linked to lifestyle factors such as poor food and insufficient exercise, has skyrocketed. It has an effect on the body's ability to regulate blood sugar levels.

A number of factors contribute to the sudden emergence of pandemics, including:

• Travel and Globalisation: As more people travel and connect across borders, hazardous diseases are rapidly spreading over the world. As cities get denser and more populated, conditions such as inadequate sanitation, overcrowding, and limited access to healthcare become more conducive to disease transmission.

• Environmental Changes: Environmental factors such as deforestation, climate change, and human encroachment on natural habitats can disrupt ecosystems and contribute to the transfer of diseases from animals to humans.

• Infrastructure for global health: Due to gaps in healthcare systems, a lack of finance, and limited access to healthcare in some locations, effective pandemic detection, response, and control are challenging.

To address these concerns and mitigate the effects of impending pandemics, governments, international organisations, communities, and individuals must prioritise public health initiatives, invest in healthcare infrastructure, encourage the development of dispersed residential properties, and promote global cooperation.

We should all share the responsibility of taking proper care of our own communal areas, particularly as communities. Because we are the ones who limit these places, it is in our best interests to ensure that we build heaven on earth in our own worlds while also working together to revitalise family businesses and local economies by utilising local talent, professionals, and experts.

Similar to a relay race, knowledge is being imparted. These abilities can be honed, taught, and learned. The more we care for ourselves and do not rely only on the government, the more we will respect, value, and love the environment in which we live. Communities that know one another look out for one another; this approach would help to reduce crime.

Victor Schauberger developed the log flume transportation system based on his studies and observations of the shape of an egg. In addition, he observed a snake moving in a double spiral motion alongside a rapid river.

Victor noticed that by adding counter-counter-curves to the walls of the flume, he could make the logs twist in the water like a snake in water, avoiding clogs as they moved down the dam.

This wavelike movement, this vertical and horizontal curve choreography. The oval shape of the egg led Victor to build the dam wall at the flume's base. His unique design prevented a buildup of water pressure, which would have decreased its mobility and power.

Although the body has its own methods for maintaining pH levels, some people believe that certain foods can help to maintain a more alkaline environment. Natural foods that are commonly thought to be alkalising include the following:

Leafy greens: Alkaline and nutrient-dense foods such as spinach, kale, Swiss chard and collard greens.

Cruciferous vegetables: such as broccoli, cauliflower, Brussels sprouts, and cabbage, are alkalising and high in nutrients.

Citrus fruits: Although citrus fruits are naturally acidic, they have an alkalising effect on the body once metabolised. Some examples include lemons, limes, and grapefruits.

Cucumbers: Because cucumbers are hydrating and have alkaline properties, they are a refreshing alternative for maintaining pH balance.

Avocados are alkalising and high in nutrients. They also provide healthy fats that support overall health.

Almonds: Almonds are a nut that creates alkakine and can be consumed as a snack or added to meals to provide additional nutrition.

Herbal teas: Chamomile, peppermint, and ginger are a few alkaline herbal beverages that can assist support a more balanced pH.

It's vital to remember that when compared to the body's internal regulating systems, these foods have little effect on pH levels.

Instead of focusing solely on individual meals to alkalise the body, the emphasis should be on overall dietary patterns.

Maintaining a well-balanced diet comprised of a variety of nutrient-dense foods is always recommended to enhance overall health and wellbeing.

Your body is your most significant asset... in all of our lives!

And the best key to your health is what we consume. So let's have a look at that. Vegetarians eat grains, legumes, nuts, seeds, vegetables, and fruit. Organic dairy goods such as cheese and milk (produced with vegetable and fruit rennet) and fresh organic eggs are also popular. The average vegetarian is more likely to consume the daily required amount of fruits and vegetables.

And prefers to cook with healthy plant oils like olive, coconut, or sesame...rather than animal fat. Some people use clarified oil, such as ghee. Vegan diets are considered healthful because they are plant-based and include beans, pulses, nuts, and seeds but do not include dairy. The vegan diet is also thought to lower the risk of ailments such as obesity, hypertension, cholesterol, diabetes, and possibly heart disease.

In the meanwhile, a Pescatarian diet consists solely of fish and vegetables.

Grains and legumes, as well as a moderate amount of dairy, provide the benefits of what is commonly referred to as a "Mediterranean diet." Which can provide a tasty balanced meal if you stick to organic fish...and please avoid factory farmed fish, which can be hazardous.

All types of food and drinks are parts of a diet.

The ideal diet depends on how your body responds to the food you choose to eat. It also depends on the nutrients most required by your immune system to stay in balance. Your body type is also key. As we learn from the development of the body, that the food you eat becomes you... So does the food you eat love you back?

Chapter 6: Types of Diet

A diet can consist of any type of food or drink.

The optimum diet for you is determined by your body's reaction to the foods you choose to eat. It also depends on the nutrients that your immune system requires the most in order to stay in balance. Your body type is also significant. As we can see from the development of the body, you are what you consume... Does the food you eat return your affection?

A diet is the kind of food and drink that a society or a person usually eats and drinks regularly.

And dieting means sticking to a special type of food to which a person restricts themselves. Usually for the purpose of loosing weight. And conversely sometimes for the purpose of gaining weight. So an ideal diet is the one that enables you to maintain a healthy weight according to your body type and built. Ensuring balance balance between the body and mind.

Eating inevitably means you consume various types of life changing produce. Food and nutrients which in turn affect your digestion. All food and plants, nuts, grains, vegetables and fruit and even life itself comes from Mother Earth. As well as meat and fish. And whatever you eat builds your body. Every meal, snack or drink, transforming your very being.

The simpler the food you eat, for example vegetables, fruit, plants, seeds, nuts, etc. the easier they become part of your body. However as these foods themselves posses no emotions, they have no specific impact on your emotional state.

The more complex the food, such as rabbit, pheasant, geese, pig, poultry such as chicken, turkey, as well as ducks, pheasants, and partridge, beef and fish, the more distinct this gets. because animals, like humans, have emotions.

And new research shows that the cows used to manufacture your regular burger are highly sentient, intelligent individuals with distinct personalities. They actually have colourful, passionate personalities.

Humans are the only creatures that ingest milk from other mammals. comparable to goat or cow milk. Human milk is not consumed by goats and cows.

Most people never give this any thought. Current research, however, indicates that ingesting milk from other mammals is detrimental to humans.

Most societies do not butcher and eat dogs because they have strong emotions and, like people, create emotional bonds with those around them. As a result, because we now know that animals have emotions, more people are choosing not to eat meat, which normally requires preparation.

Furthermore, we now know that eating food as raw as possible reduces the risk of disease by at least 40 to 50 percent. And 'Yes,' some items must be cooked before they can be eaten. However, much more food is nutritious when taken raw, which is why we prepare salads and eat veggies in their natural, unadulterated state.

As a result, you can increase the amount of nutrition entering your metabolism while remaining healthy in terms of weight and age. The biggest advantage of raw food is its light weight, which indicates how easy it will be to digest. This provides the body with energy for the day.

Mind the Body and Food's Relationship to Chakras

The connection between food and the chakras stems from the notion that everything is made out of energy. And all life in the universe is made up of energy.

Energy is the vital power that permits various biological activities and supports live creatures in the context of life and all living things.

Energy is the ability to conduct labour or effect change, and it is essential in all parts of life, from cellular processes to ecosystem functioning.

All biological things, according to scientific understanding, are made up of atoms and molecules that interact and exchange energy. These interactions entail the transfer and transformation of energy in a variety of forms, including chemical energy, thermal energy, electrical energy, and others.

Energy is used by living organisms for growth, reproduction, mobility, metabolism, and other biological activities required for survival.

Furthermore, the idea that all living things are constituted of energy is strongly related to a knowledge of the universe's interconnection. Everything in the universe is made up of energy at its most basic level.

This concept is consistent with scientific principles such as energy conservation, which states that energy can only be transformed from one form to another and cannot be created or destroyed.

From a metaphysical or spiritual stance, the idea that all living things are formed up of one energy fosters a sense of connectedness and oneness among all beings.

This concept is commonly associated with philosophical and religious systems that emphasise the interdependence of all things. It indicates that all living things are linked by the same underlying energy or life force in a greater cosmic web.

Although it may go beyond scientific explanations, this approach provides a framework to explore the inherent interdependence and shared essence of all living things. It has the potential to instil compassion, wonder for life, and awareness of our relationship with the natural world.

Man and woman were created in the image of the infinite wisdom, who also ordered that they must reproduce and multiply. He also created nature, which provides man with sustenance, nourishment, and healing in the form of food, seeds, plants, spices, and herbs.

This is a general overview of the chakras and the foods associated with each one:

Muladhara (Root Chakra): The root chakra is associated with feelings of security, stability, and grounding. Protein-rich foods like beans and lentils, as well as root vegetables like carrots, potatoes, and beets, are said to help balance this chakra.

Svadhisthana (Sacral Chakra): is associated with creativity, sentiments, and sensuality. Foods with bright orange colours, such as oranges, mangoes, and sweet potatoes, as well as nuts, seeds, and healthy fats, are said to promote the sacral chakra.

Manipura (The Solar Plexus Chakra): is associated with self-confidence, digestion, and personal power. Foods with a yellow tinge, such as lemons, bananas, whole grains, and spices like ginger and turmeric, are said to nourish this chakra.

Water makes up around 60% of the human body.

The specific proportion can vary depending on factors such as age, gender, body composition, the natural food you eat contains water. As well as the natural beverages like herbal tea, all together form the total amount of water you consume per day. And, overall health counts. Water promotes digestion, maintains body temperature, and transports nutrients to cells. Water aids in many other important functions, such as joint lubrication.

It's critical to stay hydrated throughout the day by drinking plenty of water and other beverages. Although it is typically recommended to drink 8 cups (64 ounces or 2 litres) of water every day, everyone's needs differ.

Some biological systems, like the human immune system, Mother Earth, and water, have the ability to self-regulate. Human health is dependent on having access to safe drinking and bathing water.

Water may provide us with life support, but we do not completely benefit from it because of the harsh and artificial manner in which it is delivered to us.

Demystifying the Myth of Drinking 8 Cups of Water Per Day

There is no truth or natural law that requires us to consume 8 glasses of water per day. If you listen to your body, you will be able to tell when you are thirsty. Because the body's mechanism is incredibly sophisticated, it warns you before you become dehydrated.

Calories, the unit of energy comparable to body heat, affect your water intake.

The water your body uses to stay hydrated is a combination of clean water and water from organic vegetables and fruit that you consume on a daily basis.

Over-hydration produces moisture in your spleen, affecting your body's fire energy and causing water retention. As a result, oedema develops.

The fire energy in your body moves water and blood. Drinking water even when you are not thirsty generates stress in the heart and kidneys, which can lead to heart and kidney failure over time.

Your body is your subconscious mind, and your body type dictates how much water you need. People with cold spectrum body types tend to consume less water than those with warm spectrum body types.

Your daily physical activities also contribute to your body's need for water. Simply listening to your body, you will know when it's time - drink clean water from a glass not a plastic bottle. In almost all plastic products and or containers in the world, have BPA, Bisphenol A, bps, and phthalates and many other dangerous compounds.

Plastic Containers Cause Chronic Diseases

Never eat or drinking from plastic containers, especially when the plastic is hot at room or higher temperature. And particularly when the plastic container has been exposed to the high heat of the sun whilst in your car. Also avoid covering up your food with plastic wraps.

The chemicals contained in the plastic will mess-up your insulin, which cause the demise of your endocrine system - Astrogen, glands which secret hormones into your blood.

Plastic causes weight gain, infertility, Polycystic Ovary Syndrome (PCOS), Diabetes type 2, and the demise of Progesterone and Testosterone in men.

Never give your child plastic toys, human beings are not meant to eat from or babies to chew on plastic, it leads to obesity and the risk of cancer.

Water is Life, and Life is Water.

By the time the water reaches our homes, it has been through a journey that resembles a straight jacket, and its nutrients have been violently removed. I've highlighted a few benefits of water for us below.

Hydration: It is vital to consume clean water in order to stay hydrated, as this is required for all biological functions.

Water aids in the evacuation of waste products and toxins from the body, in addition to aiding digestion, vitamin absorption, and body temperature regulation.

Clean water is vital for meal digestion and nutrient absorption. It assists in the breakdown and dissolving of nutrients, allowing them to enter cells and be used in a number of biological processes.

Drinking enough of water supports intestinal health. It reduces the chances of constipation and other digestive issues by encouraging regular bowel movements and softening the stool.

Clean water is vital for kidney health since it aids in the removal of waste and toxins from the blood. Drinking plenty of water can help you avoid urinary tract infections and kidney stones

Muscle and Joint Health: Drinking plenty of fresh water will help keep your joints and muscles in good condition. Water aids in the delivery of oxygen and nutrients to muscles while also cushioning and lubricating joints for smooth movement.

Skin Health: Bathing and drinking in clean water is beneficial to your skin. With appropriate hydration, the skin can be kept moisturised, supple, and more elastic. It can also help the body remove waste and toxins through sweat, resulting in clearer and healthier-looking skin.

Clean water contributes to the body's natural cleansing processes.

It helps in comprehensive detoxification by flushing waste, metabolic by products, and toxins out of organs and tissues.

Overall Happiness: Drinking clean water and staying hydrated have an impact on overall health, energy levels, and cognitive performance. It improves mental clarity, concentration, and attention.

Clean water helps to maintain personal hygiene by removing filth, sweat, and microorganisms from the skin during a bath. Bathing in clean water can help reduce skin infections and promote overall hygiene and comfort by keeping the skin healthy and clean.

It is critical to remember that the purity and quality of water may vary depending on the source and location. It is critical to have access to safe drinking water, and it is prudent to follow local water safety norms and laws.

If there are safety concerns about the water, it may be necessary to employ water filtration systems or seek alternative sources of pure water to obtain the most health advantages. I'll add one more item.

A healthy mind goes hand in hand with a healthy body.

You, too, have gone through experiences that have enriched your life. Whether you're a mother, expecting a child, or want to establish a family.

I hope this book inspires and motivates you to make the best decision for your health. With your enthusiasm for life and a deeper understanding of what causes you joy, perhaps you will be able to adopt healthy habits that will benefit future generations, including your children, Take each day as it comes and maintain consistency. Furthermore, I hope everything goes well for you, and I appreciate you.

The energy within living organisms is utilised for growth, reproduction, movement, metabolism, and other biological processes necessary for sustaining life.

Moreover, the concept of all living things being made of energy is closely related to the understanding of the interconnectedness of the universe. At a fundamental level, everything in the universe is made up of energy.

This concept aligns with scientific principles, such as the conservation of energy, which states that energy cannot be created or destroyed but only transformed from one form to another.

From a metaphysical or spiritual perspective, the idea that all living things are one energy advocates a sense of interconnectedness and unity among all beings and nature.

My final word

A healthy body exists in a healthy mind as everything begins in the mind

This was one of the profound lessons I learnt from my father. Among many other lessons I learnt from him, was that the purpose of eating is not for filling up the belly. Rather, mainly for nourishing the body so as to maintain a balanced level of energy between the body and mind.

Added to that he said, always remember; 'books are the best man's friend' ...and last but not least, putting your lessons into action helps you grow spiritually, intellectually and creatively.

These lessons became a foundation upon which I formulated my philosophy. Based on the lessons my father learnt from his Chinese Master who trained him as a martial artist in Karate and Judo. And his enthusiasm for spiritual growth helped him cross paths with Maharishi Mahesh's meditation teachings, whose workshops we had the privilege to attend. This was the footing upon which I formulated my philosophy for a health lifestyle.

We have all had experiences that have been a positive force in our lives. Whether you are a mum, or a mother to be or are planning to start your family. I hope this book will encourage you to choose the best path for a healthy lifestyle. When you define what make you feel the happiness within you, you will be strong enough to follow an unwavering code of conduct regarding your health that will also benefit your children.The children are our future, therefore they deserve a good start in life.

Thank you... I wish you well !

Acknowledgements

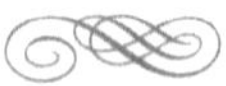

There are numerous people I would like to thank. People who have served as my mentors and have assisted me in better understanding how modern agriculture and food severely impact our mental and physical health. I am grateful to all of my teachers, both those who have taught me in the past and those who are currently teaching me.

I am always be grateful to my wonderful spouse, Barney Edwards, for his love, support, and companionship. Ntuthuko Lolly Gumbi, my most adored daughter, for her love, support, and wit. Lathitha, my most adorable grandchild, inspires me with her sense of humour and sunflower smile. My loving parents, Nonceba, my late mother, and my most cherished farther Mandlesilo Gumbi, for their love and support. And my late grandfather, James Nduna Gumbi, whose love of writing and entrusting me with his manuscripts opened up a part of me I never knew existed after reading them. Until I attempted to put my beliefs and experiences on living a truly holistic lifestyle on paper. Teaching me the value of how each person who plays a significant role in our life adds another depth to the fabric of who we are. As a result, he is still alive in me. And now is the time in my life when I feel ready to share my experiences and expertise, highlighting ways to preserve the benefits of a balanced and healthy lifestyle. Putting nature and food at the heart of excellent health. Bringing happiness and encouragement into our life. When we are in a state of love, we are pure. Sharing and spreading love is caring...which is exactly what I intend to accomplish with this book!

About the Author

As a little girl I was trained as a gymnast by my Father.

A Personal Trainer, Marshal Arts and Gymnastics Coach.

There was one thing my Father was super strict about ...my diet.

He would say ...*"never ever forget ...you are what you eat* !"

It's one of the most important lessons I ever learnt.

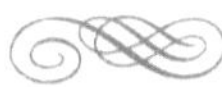

Ruby Gumbi-Edwards was born in South Africa where she was educated.

After her studies, Ruby embarked on a successful career in the corporate world of Banking, HR and Marketing. After meeting her husband, she joined the film industry as a Producer.

When she settled with her husband in London, she transitioned into the art industry, following her bliss, she worked for prominent artists as a photography colourist, archivist, buyer and curator.

Driven by her innate desire to inspire and empower others to live healthy and fulfilling lives, Ruby continues to be a beacon of inspiration, sharing her expertise and passion for holistic wellness through personal training and sharing her knowledge on online platforms.

Today, Ruby continues to be a beacon of inspiration, sharing her expertise and passion for holistic wellness through personal training and sharing her knowledge on online platforms.

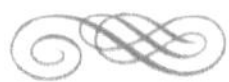

Don't miss out!

Visit the website below and you can sign up to receive emails whenever Ruby Gumbi-Edwards publishes a new book. There's no charge and no obligation.

https://books2read.com/r/B-A-CZSS-NJDMC

BOOKS 2 READ

Connecting independent readers to independent writers.

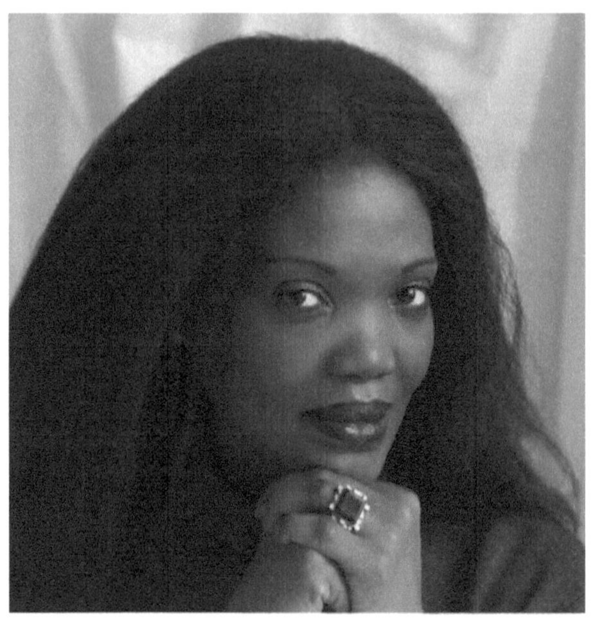

About the Author

About the Author

As a little girl I was trained as a gymnast by my Father.

A Personal Trainer, Marshal Arts and Gymnastics Coach.

There was one thing my Father was super strict about ...my diet.

He would say ...*"never ever forget ...you are what you eat* !"

It's one of the most important lessons I ever learnt.

Ruby Gumbi-Edwards was born in South Africa where she was educated.

After her studies, Ruby embarked on a successful career in the corporate world of Banking, HR and Marketing. After meeting her husband, she joined the film industry as a Producer.

When she settled with her husband in London, she transitioned into the art industry, following her bliss, she worked

for prominent artists as a photography colourist, archivist, buyer and curator.

Driven by her innate desire to inspire and empower others to live healthy and fulfilling lives, Ruby continues to be a beacon of inspiration,

sharing her expertise and passion for holistic wellness through personal training and sharing her knowledge on online platforms.

Today, Ruby Gumbi-Edwards continues to be a beacon of inspiration, sharing her expertise and passion for holistic wellness through personal training and sharing her knowledge on online platforms.